HEART DISEASE HERBAL TEAS

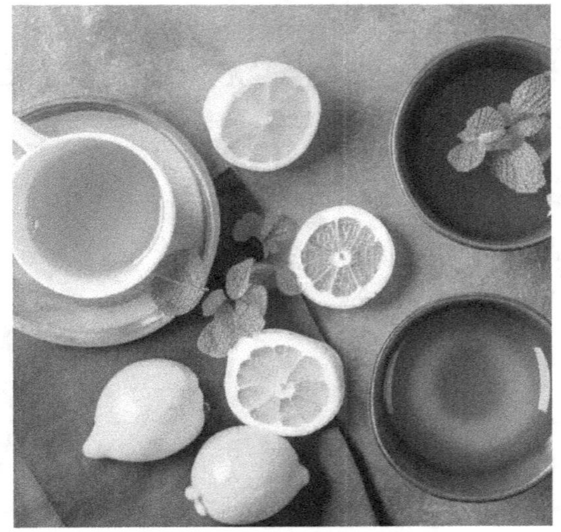

The Best Natural Tea Remedies

Jessica Murray

Dear Reader,

Thank you for the purchase. I hope you enjoy and love it, would you consider dropping an honest feedback/review, I will appreciate that and you can contact me using JessicaMurrayDietHelp@gmail.com if you have any questions, I will gladly respond

Table of Contents

INTRODUCTION

Eighteen months ago, John received a heart condition diagnosis. He was given prescriptions to take home, and his prognosis was not promising. He was advised to exercise frequently, make an effort to eat healthily, and reduce his salt intake—all things he had already tried and failed to achieve.

John came upon a book of herbal teas for heart problems one evening while searching the internet for home cures. He was sceptical because he was aware that this kind of event was unusual, but he chose to give it a shot.

The herbal drinks became a part of John's everyday regimen. He made himself a cup of the suggested tea every morning and every evening, and within a few days he could tell a change. When he drank the tea, his chest felt lighter, and he was able to go farther on his daily walks.

After 18 months, John's perspective has significantly changed. His doctor has taken him off the majority of his medications, and thanks to the herbal teas and healthy lifestyle, his blood pressure and cholesterol levels are better than they've ever been.

John continues to drink the herbal tea as part of his daily routine and is amazed by how well it has worked to manage his heart problems. His belief in the effectiveness of herbal teas and their therapeutic advantages has grown.

HERBAL TEAS

Hibiscus Tea

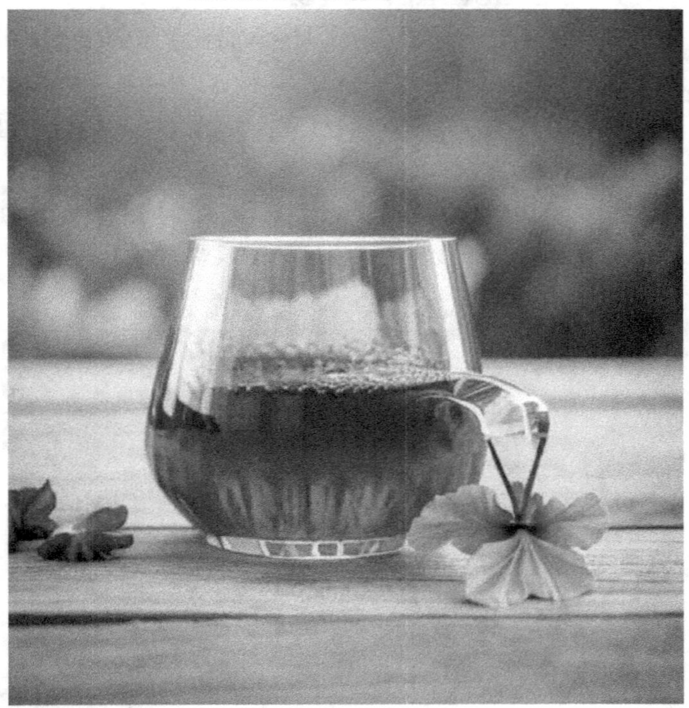

Ingredients:
- 1 cup of hot water
- 1-2 teaspoons of hibiscus flowers

Instructions:
- Fill a mug with boiling water and add hibiscus flowers.
- Steep for 10 minutes, then drain and, if required, sweeten to taste.

Hawthorn Tea

Ingredients:

- 1 cup boiling water
- 1 teaspoon dried hawthorn berries

Instructions:

- Add hot water to the mug with the hawthorn berry
- Steep for 10 minutes, then drain and, if required, sweeten to taste.

Yarrow Tea

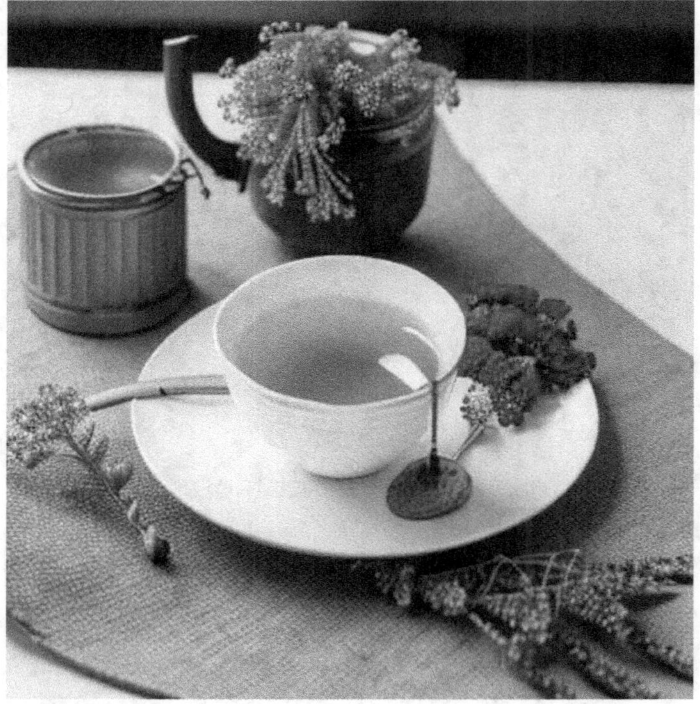

Ingredients:

- 1 cup of hot water, 1 teaspoon of dried yarrow flowers

Instructions:

- Add hot water to the mug with the yarrow flowers
- Steep for 10 minutes, then drain and, if required, sweeten to taste.

Motherwort Tea

Ingredients:

- 1 teaspoon dried motherwort leaves,
- 1 cup hot water

Instructions:

- Add hot water to the mug with the motherwort leaves.
- Steep for 10 minutes, then drain and, if required, sweeten to taste.

Dandelion Root Tea

Ingredients:

- 1 cup hot water,
- 2 teaspoons dried dandelion root

Instructions:

- Add hot water to the mug with the dandelion root.
- Steep for 10 minutes, then drain and, if required, sweeten to taste.

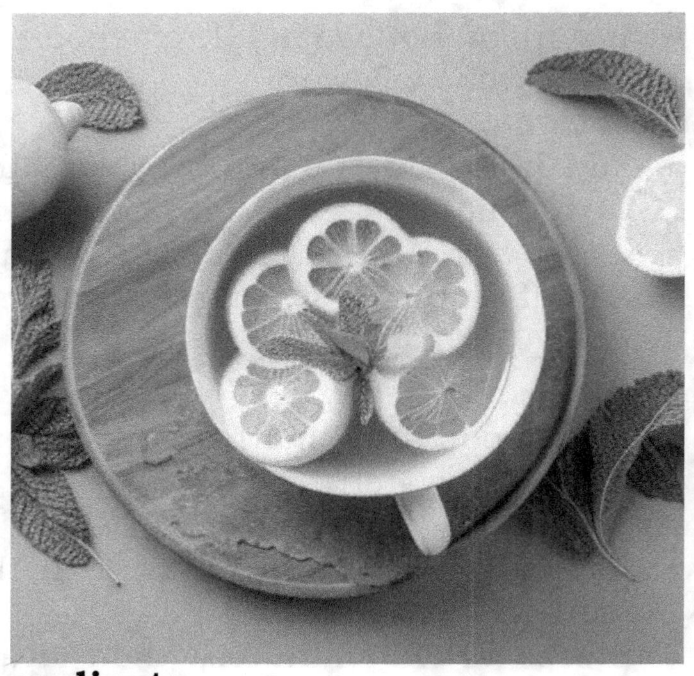

Ingredients:

- 1 teaspoon dried lemon balm leaves and 1 cup boiling water.

Instructions:

- Put some lemon balm leaves in a mug, then fill it with hot water.
- Steep for 10 minutes, then drain and, if required, sweeten to taste.

Green Tea

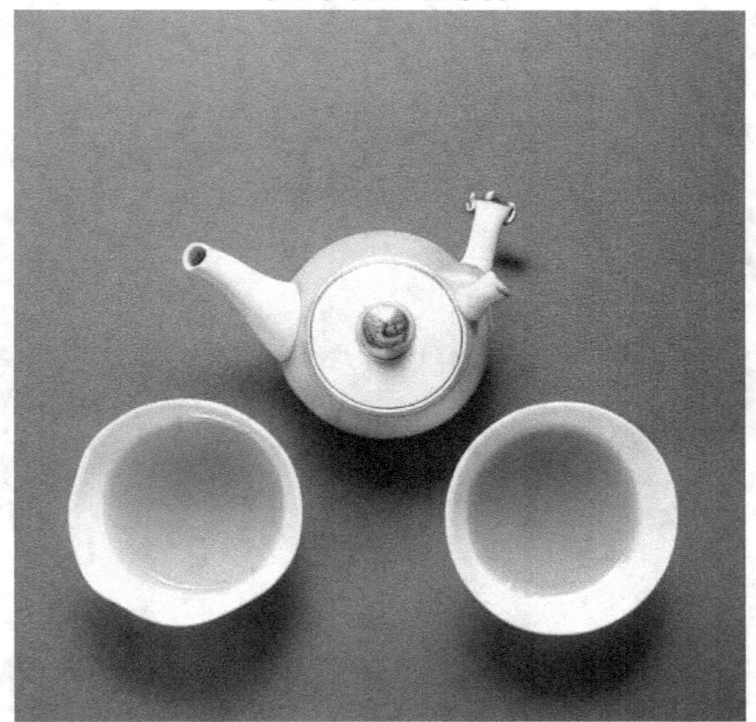

Ingredients:

- 1 cup of hot water, 1-2 tablespoons of green tea leaves

Instructions:

- Add hot water to the mug with the green tea leaves. Allow to steep for two to three minutes, then drain and, if desired, sweeten to taste.

Cardamom Tea

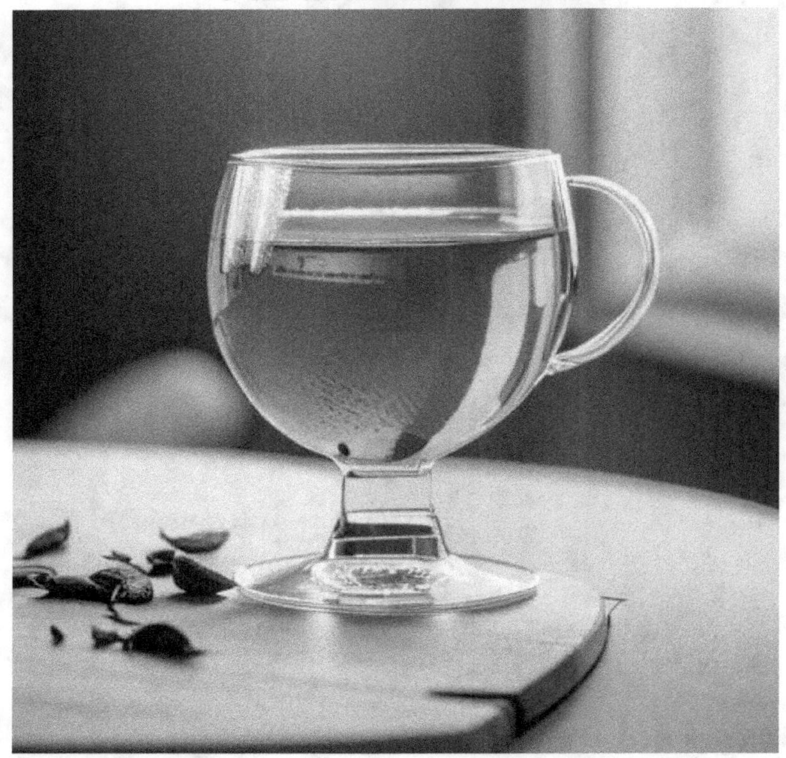

Ingredients:

- 1 cup hot water, a couple of cardamom pods

Instructions:

- Add hot water to a mug with cardamom pods inside. Steep for 10 minutes, then drain and, if required, sweeten to taste.

Ginger Tea

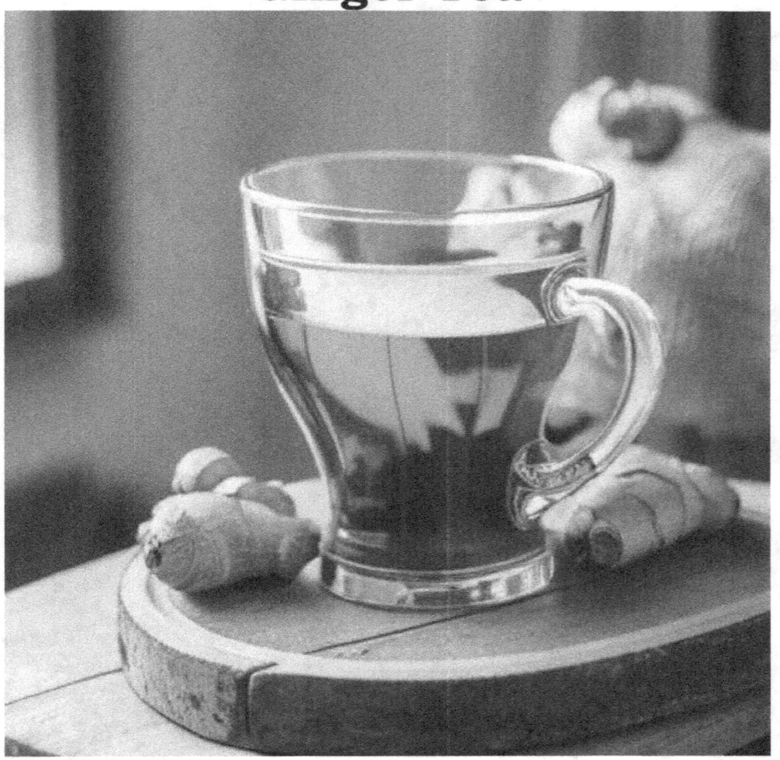

Ingredients:
- Freshly grated ginger and one cup of boiling water

Instructions:
- Add hot water to a mug with freshly grated ginger. Steep for 10 minutes, then drain and, if required, sweeten to taste.

Garlic Tea

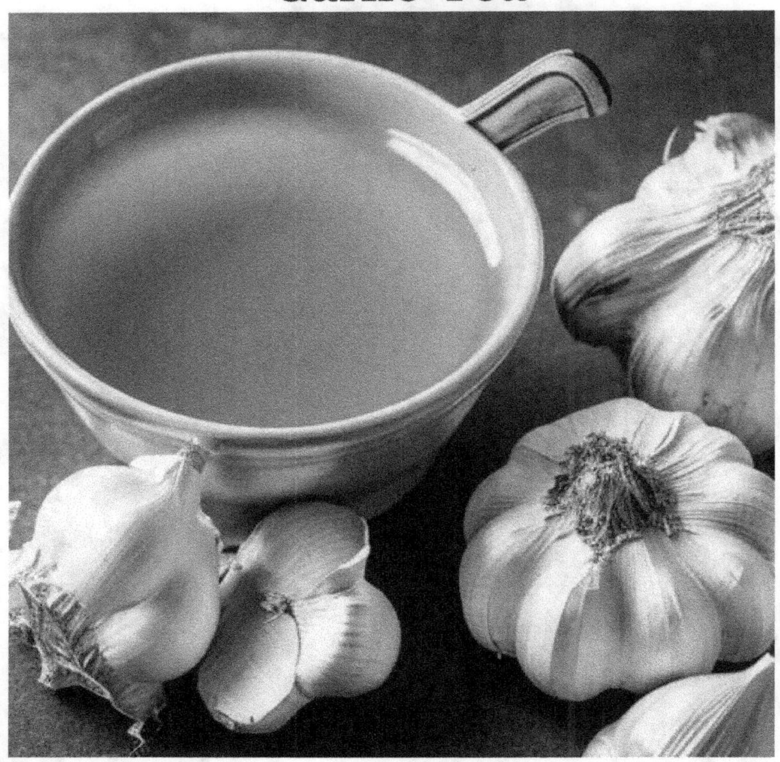

Ingredients:

- 1 cup of hot water, 1-2 garlic cloves

Instructions:

- Add hot water to a mug with garlic cloves in it. Steep for 10 minutes, then drain and, if required, sweeten to taste.

Cinnamon Tea

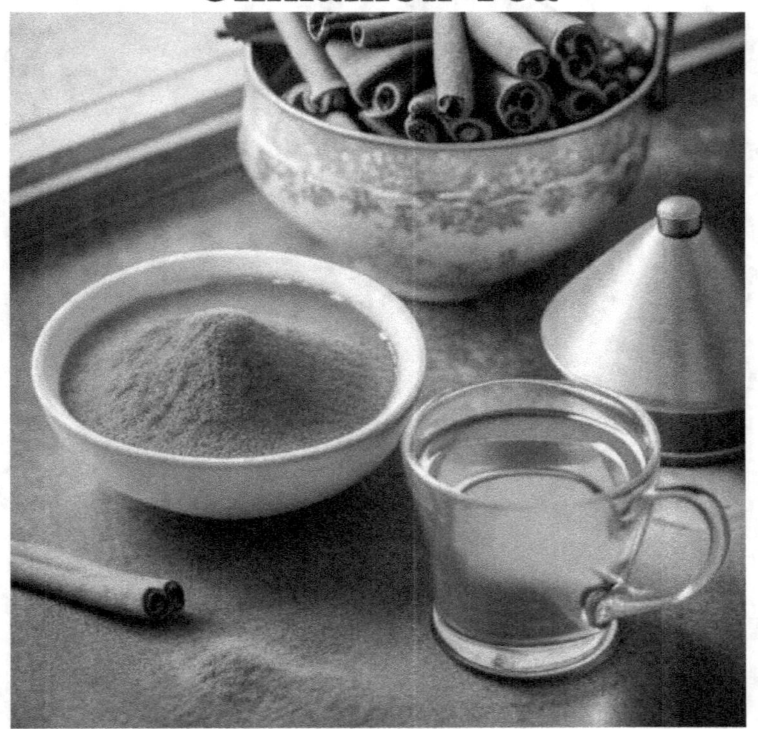

Ingredients:
- 1 cup of hot water, 2 cinnamon sticks

Instructions:
- Add hot water to the mug with the cinnamon sticks. Steep for 10 minutes, then drain and, if required, sweeten to taste.

Ginkgo Biloba Tea

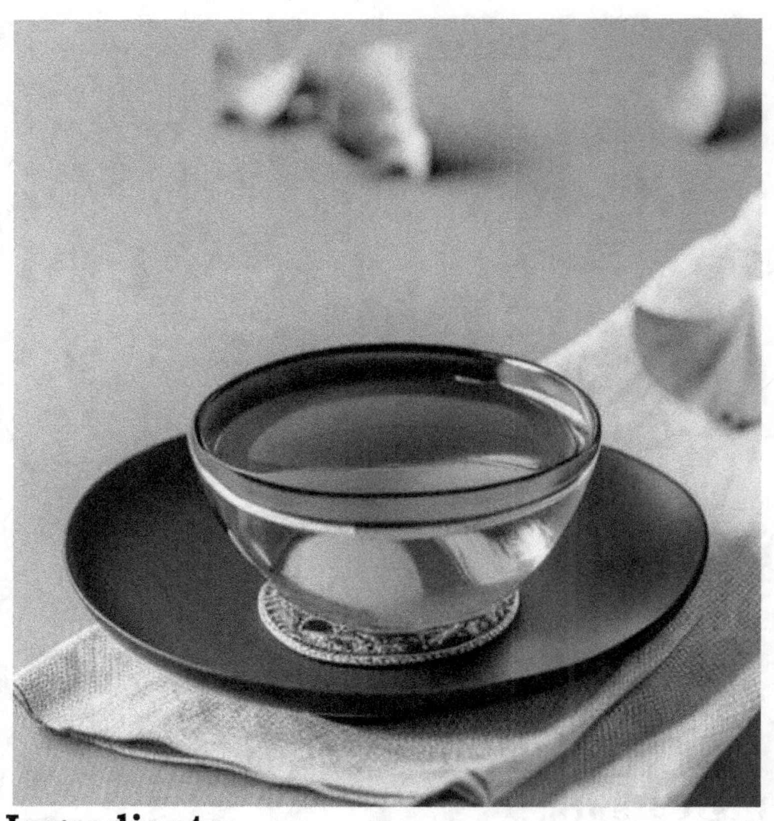

Ingredients:

- 1 cup of hot water, 2 teaspoons of dried ginkgo biloba leaves

Instructions:

- Fill a mug with boiling water and add ginkgo biloba leaves. Steep for 10 minutes, then drain and, if required, sweeten to taste.

Any Berry Tea

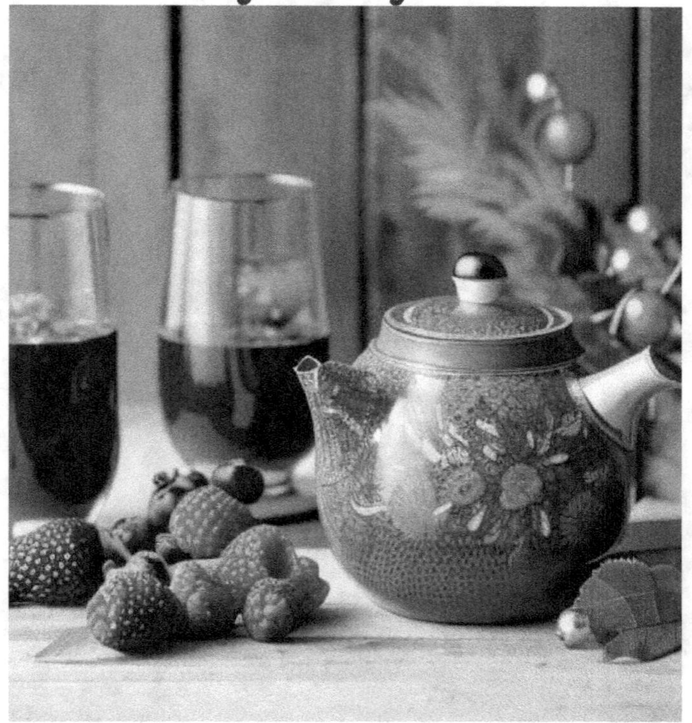

Ingredients:

- 1 cup of boiling water and 1 teaspoon of dried berries (such as cranberries, blackberries, blueberries, and raspberries).

Instructions:

- Add boiling water to a mug with dried berries in it. Steep for 10 minutes, then drain and, if required, sweeten to taste.

Oolong Tea

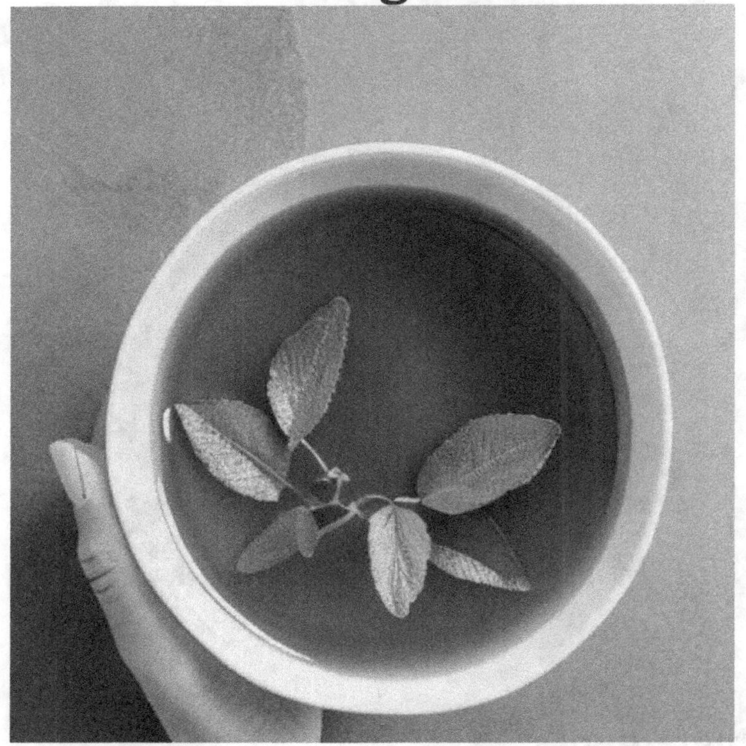

Ingredients:

- 1 cup of hot water, 1 teaspoon of oolong tea leaves

Instructions:

- Add hot water to the mug with the oolong tea leaves. Allow to steep for two to three minutes, then drain and, if desired, sweeten to taste.

Rooibos Tea

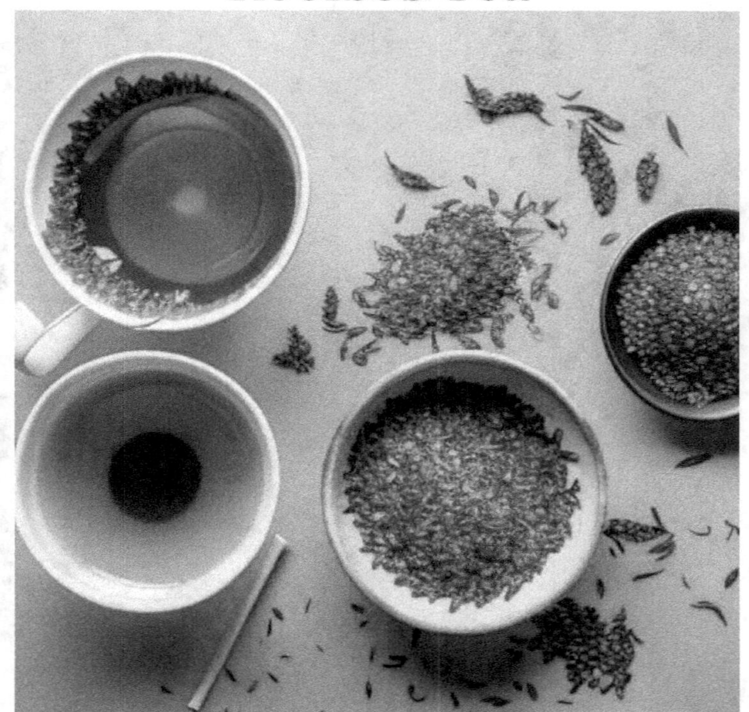

Ingredients:

- 1 cup of boiling water and 1 teaspoon of rooibos tea leaves.

Instructions:

- Add hot water to a mug with rooibos tea leaves. Steep for 10 minutes, then drain and, if required, sweeten to taste.

Rosemary Tea

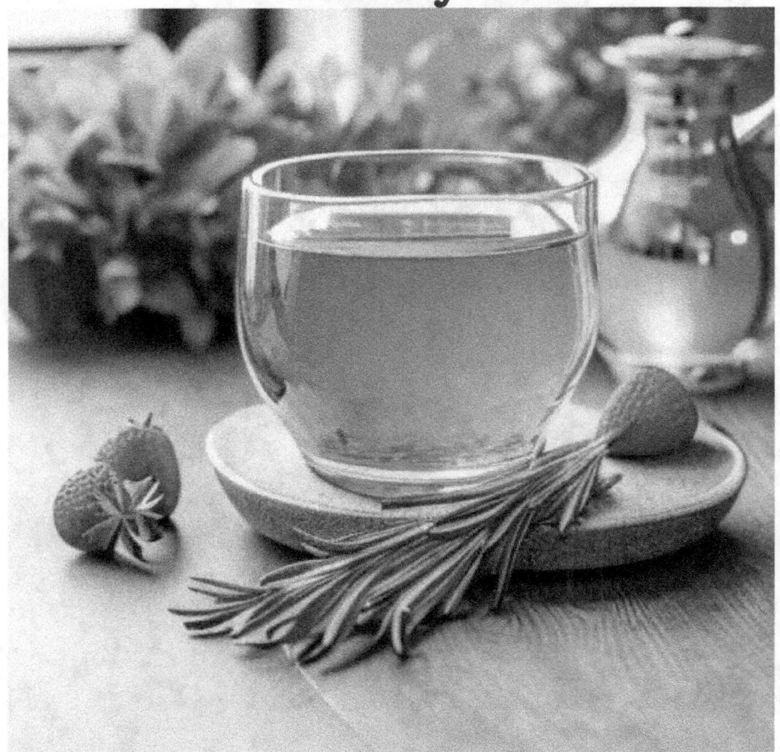

Ingredients:

- 1 teaspoon rosemary leaves, 1 cup hot water

Instructions:

- Add boiling water to a mug with rosemary leaves inside. Steep for 10 minutes, then drain and, if required, sweeten to taste.

Calendula and Rosehip Tea

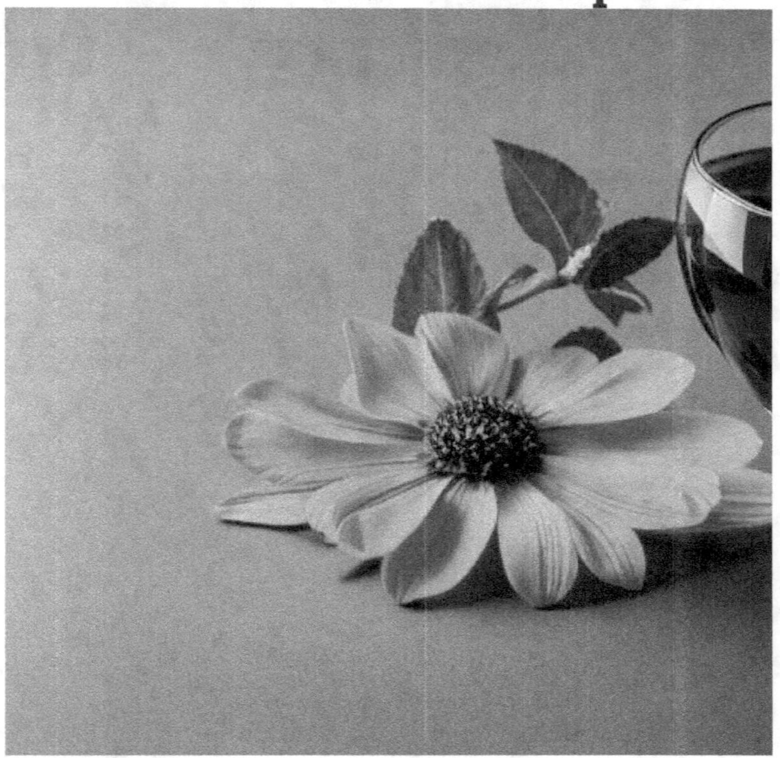

Ingredients:

- 1 cup of boiling water, 1 teaspoon each of dried rosehips and calendula flowers

Instructions:

- In a mug, combine the calendula and rosehips. Fill with boiling water. Steep for 10 minutes, then drain and, if required, sweeten to taste.

Parsley Tea

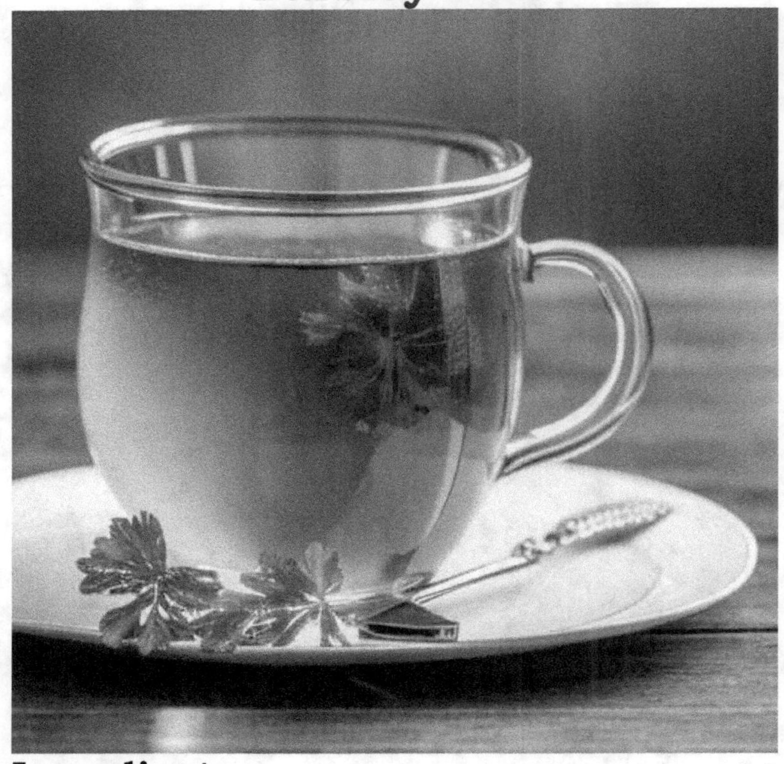

Ingredients:

- 1 teaspoon dried parsley leaves and 1 cup boiling water.

Instructions:

- Add hot water to the mug with the parsley leaves. Steep for 10 minutes, then drain and, if required, sweeten to taste.

CONCLUSION

In terms of lowering the chance of getting heart disease, drinking herbal teas can be quite beneficial. According to studies, several herbal teas can enhance circulation, lower inflammation, and cut cholesterol levels. Additionally, some herbal teas' antioxidant content can aid in preventing the free radical damage that can contribute to some types of heart disease. Teas made from herbs can be a delightful and beneficial way to strengthen the heart. Herbal teas are an easy and secure way to supplement a heart-healthy diet and lifestyle, but additional research is required.

I'm grateful that you took the time to read my book. I hope you like it and it gave you something to think about. Thank You

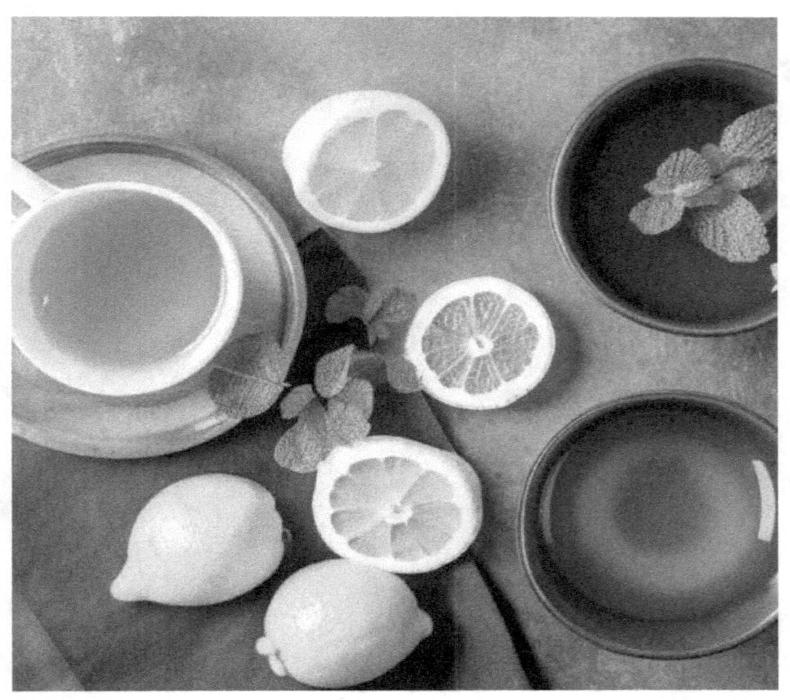